Understanding Anxiety In Relationship

A Comprehensive Guide To Overcoming Insecurity And Negative Thinking, Deal With Jealousy And Feel Secure By Uncovering The Blocks Preventing You From A Loving Union

John Myers

&

Ashley Anita Gray

Copyright - 2021 - All rights reserved.

The content contained within this book may not be reproduced, duplicated or transmitted without direct written permission from the author or the publisher.

Under no circumstances will any blame or legal responsibility be held against the publisher, or author, for any damages, reparation, or monetary loss due to the information contained within this book. Either directly or indirectly.

Legal Notice:

This book is copyright protected. This book is only for personal use. You cannot amend, distribute, sell, use, quote or paraphrase any part, or the content within this book, without the consent of the author or publisher.

Disclaimer Notice:

Please note the information contained within this document is for educational and entertainment purposes only. All effort has been executed to present accurate, up to date, and reliable, complete information. No warranties of any kind are declared or implied. Readers acknowledge that the author is not engaging in the rendering of legal, financial, medical or professional advice. The content within this book has been derived from various sources. Please consult a licensed professional before attempting any techniques outlined in this book.

By reading this document, the reader agrees that under no circumstances is the author responsible for any losses, direct or indirect, which are incurred as a result of the use of information contained within this document, including, but not limited to, - errors, omissions, or inaccuracies.

TABLE OF CONTENTS

INTRODUCTION 10

CHAPTER 1 - Conflict Resolution & Transforming Conflict .. 12
What Happens When Conflict Is Ignored 12
Boundaries 14
Agree to Disagree 16
Compromise 19
Give Conflict the Consideration It Deserves 22

CHAPTER 2 - Self Confidence 24
How Confidence Affects Every Single Part of Your Life 26
The Importance of Positivity 28
How to Increase Confidence in 5 Steps 29
Fake It Until You Make It 30
Work on Your Positivity 31
Force Yourself Out of Your Comfort Zone 31
Use Daily Affirmations 32
Look After Yourself 33

CHAPTER 3 - Worksheet and Techniques for Couples 34
Apologizing 35
Self-Reflection 36
Speak Openly, Freely, and Honestly 38
Accepting Your Partner's Influence 39

Ritualizing Mundane Things 40
Daily: 41
Weekly: 41
Monthly: 41
Annually: 42
Relationship Reassessment 43
Wish Lists 43

CHAPTER 4 - Don't Bad-Mouth Your Spouse 46
The Dangers of Trash-Talking Your Spouse 47
Secrets Get Out 48
People Try to Fix Things 49
It Isn't Fair to Them 49
The Problems Become Bigger 50
It Reinforces Negativity in A Relationship 50
Creates A Negative Image of Your Significant Other 51
It's Disrespectful 51
How to Stop Bad-Mouthing Your Spouse 52
Dodge Questions About Intimacy 52
Talk to Your Spouse About It 53
Call Them Out 54
Use Humor to Avert the Questions 54

CHAPTER 5 - Feedback: How to Give and Respond to It 56
Feedback and Your Brain 57
Offering Feedback 60
1.   Mind Your Purpose 60
2.   Focus on the Act, not the Actor 61
3.   Give a Criticism Sandwich 61
Receiving Feedback 63
1.   Build up an Immunity 63
2.   Take Time to Reflect 64
3.   Embrace Your Mistakes and Grow 64
The Bottom Line 65

CHAPTER 6 - Kindness Is the Key to Successful Communication 66

CHAPTER 7 - Grow Together 76
The Importance of Practicing Day After Day to Achieve a Mindful Relationship 79
Demystifying the Fairytales 83

CHAPTER 8 - Understanding the Impact of Trauma 86
The Trauma of the Abuse 91
CONCLUSION 94

INTRODUCTION

Thank you very much for purchasing this book.

Most toxic relationships are due to poor communication or a codependent bond. There is nothing you can do but try to resolve your relationship issues. In this book I will provide you with all the information you need to make sure you succeed in your intent. The advice you will find has been designed for those in need of urgent help, for those who want to change their situation and solve all the problems in their relationship. It will not be an easy path, you must first understand where the problems arise and what are the causes that trigger them, but with a little help from us we are sure that sooner or later you will be able to live the happy and healthy relationship you deserve.

Enjoy.

CHAPTER 1 - Conflict Resolution & Transforming Conflict

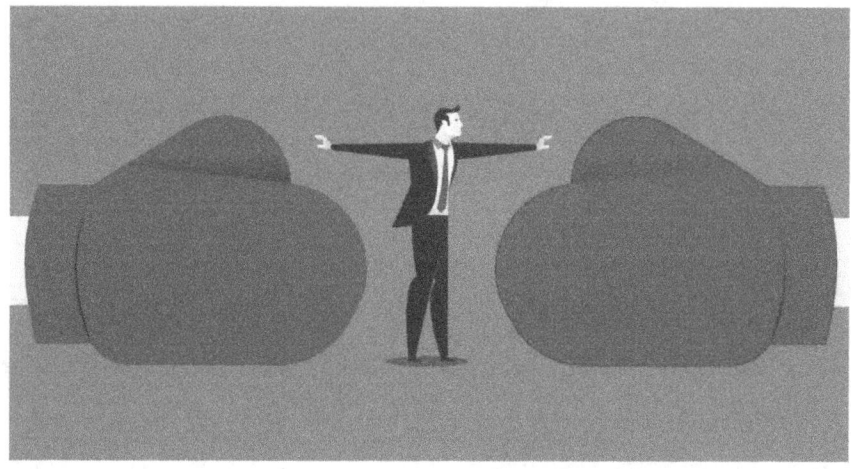

With several ways to avoid making problems worse and preventing situations at hand from getting worse, you are ready now to begin to learn conflict resolution skills.

What Happens When Conflict Is Ignored

Perhaps you feel like the easiest way to fix a conflict is to simply ignore it—if you no longer let it bother you, then it must not be important any longer, right? This is incorrect—much like ignoring an infected wound is never a proper treatment plan; ignoring conflict is the last thing you want to do.

One of the biggest reasons conflict goes ignored that one or both parties are conflict-avoidant; when conflict inevitably arises, they shut down. Instead of facing it, they sweep it under the rug and pretend it is not there to begin with. The problem with this, then, is that the rug under which you swept the last conflicts gets lumpy over time—as you sweep more and more conflict underneath it, you find yourself desperately searching for flat areas that are safe to step upon.

Those flat areas become scarcer and scarcer until your only option is to let it all out. Now, you have a myriad of problems that all need solving because you let them all build up, and that massive wall of problems is going to seem far less surmountable than if you had dealt with the problems individually as they arose.

This can lead to you deciding that the relationship is simply not worth the effort necessary to keep it alive; if the task feels like too much of an impossibility, you may instead choose to walk away. There are ways around this; however—utilizing the following conflict resolution techniques can save you from that overwhelmingly lumpy rug.

Boundaries

Perhaps the simplest way to solve conflict is to agree upon boundaries. Yes, you should have boundaries that you set when you are in a relationship with someone else. These boundaries ensure that you are being respected and honored in the way you deserve, and when you and your partner talk about which boundaries you want to set, you and your partner both know where the line is.

By agreeing to each other's boundaries, regardless of how much you may want to resist them, you acknowledge what you have to do to avoid further conflict.

For example, perhaps you have a boundary that you want to be honored— maybe you want to ensure that your partner never says something to imply that you are responsible for all housework, even jokingly. If you never tell your partner that is one of your hard limits, he has no way to know that doing so will anger you so much. He may joke, and then you find yourself in a huge conflict. You can then solve that conflict by making your boundary known. Explain why that bothers you and why you want it to be a hard limit, and acknowledge that your partner says he will avoid doing so again. It is the resolution you need in your conflict, and it will also help you avoid conflict in the future.

Agreeing to respect a boundary that is laid out in front of you is one of the easiest ways to end a conflict, especially when an apology joins it. Remember, just because your partner has a boundary that you do not necessarily agree with is not less legitimate because it is irrelevant to you.

Likewise, it is okay for you and your partner to have conflicting boundaries in regards to yourself. Perhaps you are not okay with your partner waking you up at night for intimacy, but your partner is okay with being woken up. You don't want to be woken up, but waking up your partner is not hypocritical—you can have different preferences without yours being illegitimatized.

Agree to Disagree

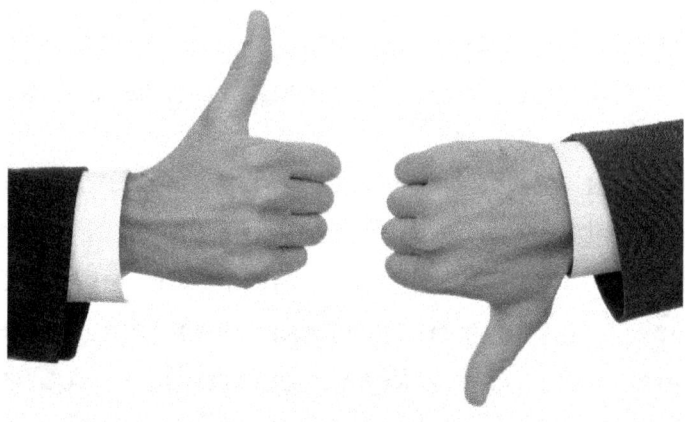

Sometimes you realize that you and your partner, no matter how much you hash out the problem or how hard you try, will never agree upon a solution. Perhaps you and your partner are fighting political views—you and your partner realize that you are both on polar opposite extremes on a particular political topic.

No matter how ridiculous you think your partner is for his position or how ridiculous your partner thinks you are for your position, neither of you are willing to budge on your positions. The more you try to make the other person see the light, the more frustrated you become.

In a situation like that, you have little choice other than agreeing to disagree. When you do this, you essentially acknowledge that you and your partner are different people.

While you may not like what your partner is insisting upon, you acknowledge that you will respect their decision and not try to change it. The key here, however, is you have to do it. You need to legitimately acknowledge and respect your partner's autonomy.

If you cannot legitimately allow your partner to believe what he believes without impacting your ability to be in your relationship, you need to stop and consider your relationship altogether. If that disagreement is something you cannot live with, that is okay, so long as you are honest about it. Remember, honesty is crucial to a relationship, and without it, your relationship will be built upon a façade of respect that, in reality, does not exist.

When you are able to agree to disagree, however, you simply stop fighting altogether with the understanding and acknowledgment of each other's positions and knowing that neither of you will ever agree upon the subject. It is not always a relationship killer, though it could be. When you agree to disagree, you are essentially saying that neither you nor the other person is willing to compromise, and you agree to it.

You agree to each of you acting independently from one another, which is not necessarily inherently unhealthy either—it is normal and healthy to have an existence outside of your partner. When you agree to disagree, your conflict melts away because you make it a non- issue.

Will it come up on occasion? Sure—maybe the upcoming election has
you once again annoyed at your partner's position.

The trick here is to recognize that since you will never agree upon the topic, you simply do not acknowledge the topic together. You know and do not like your partner's position, but have decided that it is not worth ending the relationship.

Compromise

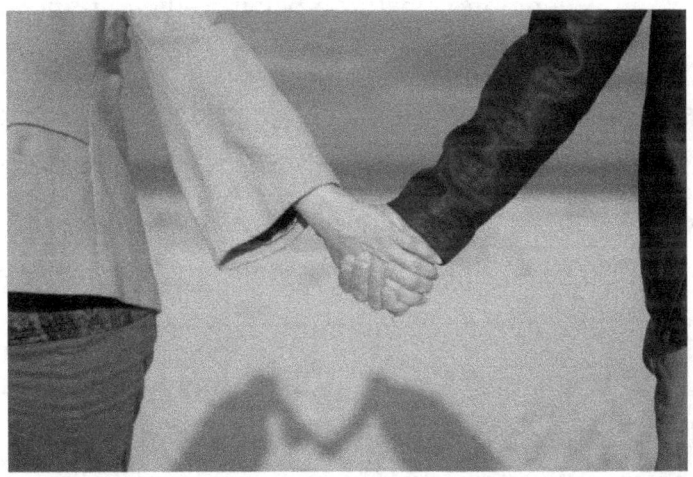

Compromise is one of the big three fundamental pillars of relationships for a reason. When you compromise, both you and your partner find yourself satisfied, at least partially. Perhaps you want to paint your living room bright teal, but your partner wants a muted grey instead.

The two of you, after realizing that both are disagree on the color, begin instead looking for colors that are acceptable to both, even if it does not bring you the same level of joy as the teal you wanted. Your partner hated the teal because it was too bright, and you hated the grey because it was too drab.

Short of painting two walls grey and two teal, you two cannot both get the color you want. Instead of bickering, you start looking at colors somewhere in the middle.

You choose muted versions of teal, and your partner sees them as an acceptable substitute because they are not bright and loud.

Suddenly, you end up with a nice, neutral teal-grey color that is neither too bright for your partner nor too drab for you. While it is not the color that really resonated with either of you, it is close enough, and something both of you can accept. Alternatively, you could agree to allow your partner to paint the bathroom that shade of red that you hated in return for you being able to paint the living room the bright teal you loved.

So long as both you and your partner both walk away with at least something you want, you have successfully compromised.

After all, your needs drive your feelings, and if you are strongly feeling something unpleasant, it is likely due to having an unmet need.

You can identify your needs with three simple steps. First, stop and try to identify what triggered the feelings.

Did something go differently than you had expected it to go? Did the unexpected result deprive you of something that you needed, whether you knew you needed it or not? If so, identify what that need that went unmet was.

This may take some introspection but should be doable. Lastly, you can meet that need by asking your partner for exactly what it is that you needed, with as much specificity as possible. In communicating what you need rather than getting into an argument, you can solve the conflict and ensure that you are meeting your needs in the future.

Give Conflict the Consideration It Deserves

The last method we will discuss in this book is learning how to consider the conflict at hand without judgment or emotion. When you consider your situation and conflict with a clear head, you can gain better insight into the situation, which can lead you to better resolve the problems you are having.

Is whatever you are arguing about actually that important to you? What will you gain by arguing with each other? If you will not gain anything, why even bother? Is agreeing to do whatever your partner is asking you to do or advocating for going to be a violation of your own core beliefs and morals?

If it is not going to violate your values, it may be worth compromising, or if it is a violation, you should try to speak to your partner to make your partner understand why you cannot do what is being requested.

Further, when you are considering the conflict, you should try to think about the point your partner is conveying. What is it that is upsetting your partner?

Can you see what your partner's position is in the argument? Is this typical for your partner? If it is atypical, what are the extenuating circumstances surrounding the event?

Stopping to consider your partner's position and comparing it to your

own will let you cue in whether you are inconsiderate or unreasonable.

23

CHAPTER 2 - Self Confidence

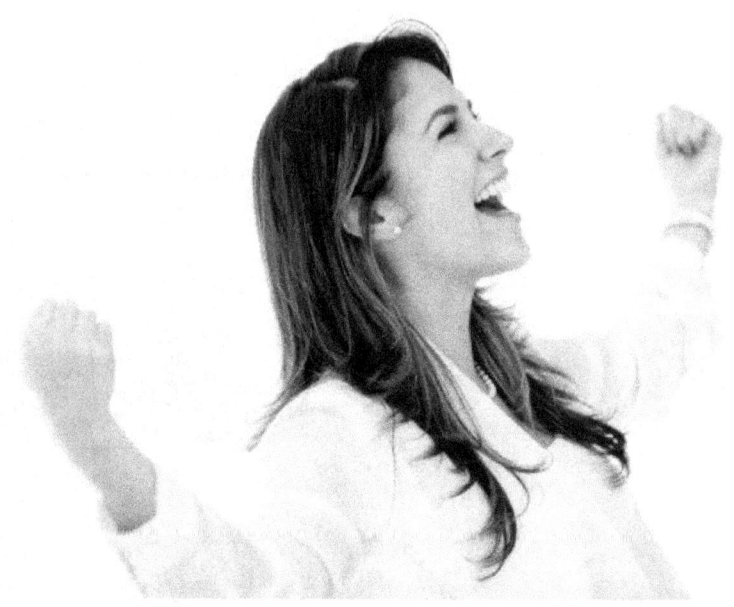

Trying to overcome any type of anxiety or fear in a relationshipis about fear, but it is also often down to a lack of confidence or self-esteem. It is the ideal breeding ground for anxiety to
continue and grow, forcing you to constantly deal with the problem daily.

Learning to build your confidence is far easier than you think. In many cases, the more you fake feeling and looking confident, the easier it comes your way! For instance, if you've ever been in a job interview and you've been extremely nervous, you were probably told to fake confidence to make the panel believe that you are far less nervous than you are. It probably worked too, whether you got the job or not!

Confidence is not something you have to work extremely hard on, but it is something you need to believe in. How will this help your relationship anxiety and insecurities? Because the more confident you are, the harder it is for those fears to work their way into your life. The harder it is for them to take control because your mind is firmly positive. Fear can only take hold when you think negatively, and part and parcel of being confident is learning to avoid negativity in the first place.

Boosting your confidence will bring you many different benefits, so let's check those out before we move on to some practical exercises to try.

How Confidence Affects Every Single Part of Your Life

Confidence is something everyone needs to be happy. As we just mentioned, when you feel confident, you feel upbeat, you feel like you can do anything, and as a result, you try more things. Doors open due to you simply having the confidence to try, and who knows where that may lead? It also means that when you are confident in yourself, you are far more likely to perhaps approach someone you like, maybe asking them out. It also means that you are far less likely to dwell on negative fears and far more likely to focus on having fun and enjoying your relationship.

Being confident is also about being healthy. When you are confident, you are positive, you are thinking clearly, and you are happy. It boosts your overall health and wellbeing and certainly does a lot to boost your mental health too. It is far harder to be depressed when you are feeling upbeat and positive, and as a result, worries won't be able to permeate your shell to the same extent. Of course, confident people still have down days and worry from time to time, but the difference is that it is very short-lived; they can work through it, shrug it off, and move on with life.

When you become more confident in life, your EQ grows too. Your ability to deal with your emotions is far greater, and you are less likely to say or do something which you might regret, such as reacting to a small thing and allowing it to turn into something far bigger in your head. It is the very situation that causes someone to perhaps accuse their partner of cheating simply because they're late home from work a few times. It does not mean that people with high EQ never have days where they worry about relationship issues, but they're able to put them into perspective and carry on with their day far easier as a result.

The Importance of Positivity

We've mentioned the P-word a few times already, so why is it so important?

When you have a negative mindset, it affects every single part of your life. You are far more prone to issues such as depression, anxiety, and stress, and you tend to become emotionally dependent on people when you should be dependent only on yourself.

When you enter into a relationship with a negative mindset, it is almost like you are waiting for it to fail, you are waiting for something to go wrong and ruin it all. It all becomes a self-fulfilling prophecy because you start to act in a way that pushes your partner away. They might start seeking solace with someone else, simply because you are so negative and down all the time, for seemingly no reason, and they can't handle it.

You are also putting yourself at risk of several health problems simply by having a negative mindset. It is because your body finds it far easier to become stressed, releasing stress hormones which stay in the body for far longer than they're supposed to. These can gradually increase your risk of heart disease and other damaging health conditions.

Aside from anything else, living a negative life is no fun!

On the other hand, if you do your best to be as positive as possible, you are far more likely to feel upbeat and happier as a result. You'll make healthier choices, you'll look for opportunities and have the confidence to take them, and all of this will add up to a life which is far more fulfilling than one which is tainted by negativity.

Think back to times when you've been around someone who was specifically negative. How did it make you feel? Drained? Negative yourself? Like you desperately needed to get out and find some positivity? That's how people feel around you when you are exuding negativity. That is not going to attract new people into your life, and it is certainly not going to boost your relationship hopes. As a result, if you enter into a relationship, it is far less likely to last.

With all of this in mind, it is important to be as positive as possible. It will help you to become a far more positive person, but a happier and more hopeful person too.

How to Increase Confidence in 5 Steps

Now you know why confidence and positive are both important in life in general, but especially in relationships, how can you work to increase your confidence levels? Here are five methods to try.

Fake It Until You Make It

A little earlier, we mentioned faking confidence, and you need to try this to see how effective it can be! Pretending to be confident when you feel far from it is a great way to build your confidence. The more confident you fake being, the more people will assume that you are. That in itself means they're going to treat you a little differently, and you'll feed off it. Over time, this will slowly boost your natural confidence levels, to the point where it all works out in reality.

Just go for it, throw away our inhibitions, and just pretend that you are confident. It does not look a certain way or sound a certain way, but it is all about the actions you give. Smile, make eye contact with people, make sure people can hear your voice, and walk with your head up and your shoulders back. You will be amazed at how quickly it changes the way you feel on the inside, and the more you do it, the more cumulative the effects will be.

Work on Your Positivity

Without going that far, however, you can work on your positivity in general. This is as easy as looking for five positive things every day and ending your day on a positive note. You can also do the same thing in the morning, by listing five positive aims for the day and doing your best to tick them off your list. It will become a competition with yourself, as you aim to tick those items off your list. As you do so, you'll feel a surge of joy with every item you tick off, and it will stick over time.

Force Yourself Out of Your Comfort Zone

The 'do something every day that scares you' adage is very true. The more you push yourself out of your comfort zone, the more you'll understand your capabilities are far greater than you realize. To date, you might have been living in a box, i.e., stuck within limitations that you've made for yourself. The world is huge; there are many things you do, and many people you can meet; why not go out there and experience it all?

Every single day, force yourself out of your comfort zone by doing one thing you wouldn't normally do. It does not have to be something that scares you, but if you want to challenge yourself in this way, go for it! If you are scared of commitment, you could use this to help you conquer your phobia, too, by taking baby steps towards your aim.

Use Daily Affirmations

We've talked about starting the day with aims and looking for positives, but how about positive affirmations. These are known confidence boosters, and over time, you'll start to believe what you are telling yourself.

The human brain learns by repetition. The more you say something to yourself and repeat it, the more you'll believe it. There is a reason why you are taught the alphabet at school by singing the song over and over again; it is because the brain catches on and commits it to a deeper, long-term memory part with repetition.

An affirmation can be anything you want it to be. It can be general, or it can be linked to a certain area of life that you want to improve. Because this is all about banishing relationship anxiety, you could make your affirmation linked to that point. Something like today, I will stay in the present and enjoy my relationship would work well. You would then repeat it three times in the morning, three times in the evening, three times at midday, and whenever you feel you need to throughout the day. The more you say it, the more you will believe it.

Look After Yourself

The very act of taking care of yourself boosts your confidence because you'll feel so much better on the inside. It means eating more healthily, making sure you get enough sleep every day, trying meditation, being mindful and living in the present, exercising regularly, having an active and a healthy social life, enjoying hobbies, learning new things regularly, and avoiding unhealthy habits, such as smoking, overeating, drinking too much, or taking drugs.

The way you feel on the inside will permeate to the outside, and you'll start to feel confident, upbeat, and able to do anything you set your mind to as a result. Your partner will also benefit from all of this, and perhaps you could focus on a healthier lifestyle together!

CHAPTER 3 - Worksheet and Techniques for Couples

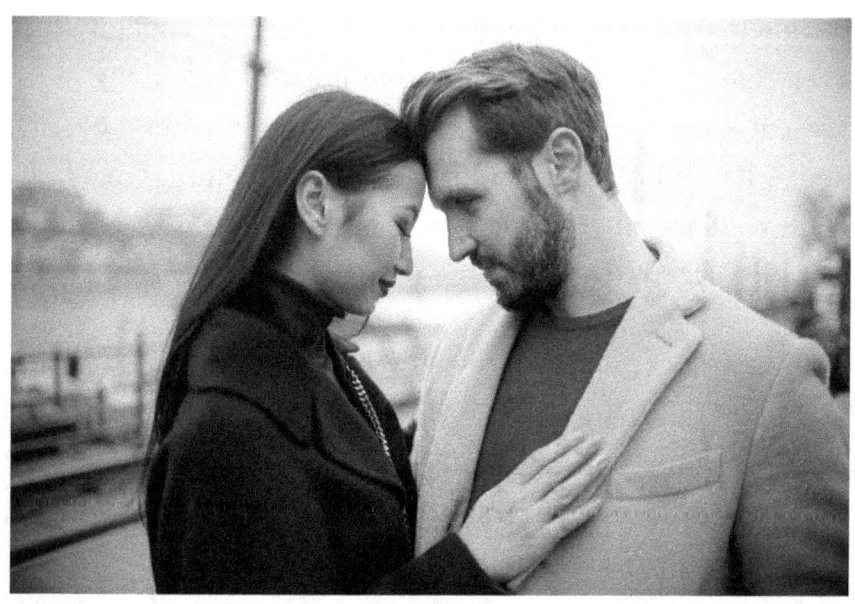

Most couples who are faced with major problems in their relationship do not realize that their relationship demands more effort, work, and dedication until it becomes too late to react to progressive conflicts and negative changes. Worksheets and techniques designed for couples who want to get the best out of their relationship are focused on exercising all key factors and qualities that make a relationship functional, happy, and healthy. To help you maintain your relationship and enhance its functionality, we share some of the top worksheets and techniques used in couples' therapy.

Apologizing

We are starting with perhaps one of the most commonly deserted acts when resolving conflicts – admitting you are wrong and apologizing for your actions, behavior, bad words, or actions. Saying I am sorry and hoping that you would be understood and forgiven is sometimes not enough, especially when it comes to major conflicts and disagreements. Let's say that you or your partner did something horrible, which affects your relationship and the way you see each other. Would a simple I am sorry to resolve the problem? Most likely, no.

That is why you need to learn how to apologize effectively so that your apology matters. An effective apology starts with acknowledging that you did something wrong while also acknowledging and recognizing that your partner is hurt and upset. You need to let your partner know that you are aware of how they feel and that you are also well aware that you are responsible for the way they feel. You need to address the problem as well, so your partner would realize that you understand why they are upset and what it is that you did wrong. This step would be explaining yourself and why you made a mistake that ended up hurting your partner. Whether you intentionally hurt your partner or unintentionally created the problem between you, you need to be honest and come clean while explaining the reason behind your actions.

Self-Reflection

Self-reflection is an important part of couple therapy, even though this exercise technique calls for individual work, which means that both partners need to participate in self-reflection, but are due to work on this exercise by themselves and without their partner's presence or influence. This technique is design to help you find gratitude and appreciation in your relationship and for your partner. We sometimes forget how lucky we are to have someone we love and who loves us back, which can backfire in losing that significant someone. Finding appreciation and gratitude for your partner will help you deepen your relationship and reflect on yourself and on everything you give and receive in your relationship. Think about the past week and every experience you had that involved your partner in those last seven days. While reflecting on your week, you need to focus on your relationship with your partner and forget about everything else as the exercise is in the process. You will create a list that will contain three different categories, each named in the following order:

- What did I receive from my partner?

- What did I give to my partner?

- Did I create a problem, and why?

- Did my partner create a problem, and why?

Once you arrange the categories of your self-reflection list, you may focus on the past week and answer the questions. For instance, under the first categories, you should write that your partner gave to you in the following week, counting on tokens of attention such as making you a coffee, packing lunch for both of you, letting you know that you are loved and appreciated, and other things that would speak in favor of a healthy relationship. Your partner should work separately on their own self-reflection list, creating the same categories as you have on your list. Under the second category, you should write everything you did for your partner in the past seven days, counting on showing care, appreciation, dedication, commitment, attention, affection, and other positive qualities that describe a healthy relationship. All couples argue and encounter disagreements every once in a while, so you need to put all disagreements and problems you believe were caused by you in the past week (if any). At the same time, the fourth category should contain the same values only concerning your partner's negative actions and behavior in the past week (if any). While working individually on your self-reflection list should help you perceive the reality of your relationship every week, comparing your lists together with your partner will help you understand how each of you perceives your relationship and everyday interactions between the two of you. Raising your awareness of what you have will help you find gratitude for your partner while listing negative experiences that took place in the near past should help you work out your problems more efficiently. Remember to be honest and trust your partner to make your relationship work. More importantly, do not take your partner for granted.

Speak Openly, Freely, and Honestly

Communication is essential; clear communication is the key to a functional relationship while speaking openly, freely, and honestly will help you reestablish and establish a deep connection and understanding between you and your partner. This exercise is created to help you work on your intimacy and sex life, need for attention, and fulfilling your partner's need for attention, as well as help you with creating a healthy environment for your relationship through communication as the main tool. We have already placed a major emphasis on how important communication in relationships is, and now we are going to present you with an effective way of removing barricades between you and your partner. In case you are struggling with being open about your needs, emotions, and thoughts, you are creating more opportunities for conflicts, misunderstandings, and disagreements. By being open and trusting that your partner will deal with openness in the same way, you are establishing a strong basis for your relationship. That way, you may come clean with any problem you think you have and show verbal appreciation to your partner.

Take action, communicate, be open, and expressing yourself might as well turn into ultimate fun times. The same goes for any other aspect of your relationship. If you feel like being hugged, you may ask your partner, do you want me to hug you? or Would you like me to hug you. When it comes to disagreements and hardships, you should as well be brave enough to state your mind and be honest, free, and open. When you feel like something has been done wrong to you, and you believe that your partner is directly responsible for the way you feel, you may state your mind and say: I do not feel that well because… or I think that what you did is wrong because… Be open, free, and honest when it comes to taking the opposite role – in cases where you are the one who's done something wrong.

Accepting Your Partner's Influence

Old habits die hard may be true, but when you are a part of a collective such as family, marriage, or a relationship, sometimes your habits need to be changed, revised, diminished and transformed. A part of this change of habits and the ways you are acting and reacting to internal and external factors will be mildly or fairly transformed without your awareness as you are sharing a relationship with your partner. However, some of your partner's influences should be accepted intentionally and with full awareness. This exercise is narrowly related to the aspect of decision making in relationships. Decision making in relationships concerns every decision that may influence your relationship, while both partners are due to make this type of decision together and within an agreement. To avoid conflict of interests, arguments, and inability to come to an agreement when trying to make a decision together, you and your partner can make a set of rules.

Ritualizing Mundane Things

This exercise is perhaps the most fun by far as you will be able to work together with your partner on creating rituals out of everyday things and activities that you will both follow up with and adopt within an agreement. Both partners may make suggestions on which activities should be shared and ritualized, i.e., done seasonally, daily, weekly, monthly, yearly. Rituals will help you make a deeper connection with your partner through romanticizing everyday activities – these activities will be the anchor of keeping up the positive dynamic in your relationship. You can make a list of all activities you and your partner would like to include. Take a look at our sample list of bonding rituals for couples.

Daily:

- Drinking coffee together in the morning
- Meeting up for lunch
- Having dinner together

Weekly:

- Going out
- Sharing a hobby
- Watching your favorite TV show
- Watching a movie
- Cooking dinner together

Monthly:

- Go on a romantic getaway weekend
- Double-date night

Annually:

- Celebrating your anniversary

- Doing something nice for each other's birthdays

You and your partner may agree to ritualize activities that both of you enjoy and appreciate, which is more than an effective way of connecting with your partner and creating pleasurable milestones on a daily, weekly, monthly, and yearly basis.

Relationship Reassessment

Reassessing your relationship and values held in the most important aspects of your relationship with your partner will help you determine which areas would use improvement and which areas are working properly. Being aware of weaknesses and strengths in your relationship will help you appreciate all the good things between you and your partner while helping you develop awareness of everything that needs to be changed to improve your relationship. You can easily reassess your relationship by creating a list based on the following pattern:

Wish Lists

Yes, making lists is an extremely effective way of taking the very first steps towards making a positive action, which is why we are making yet another list. You and your partner will once again create separate lists that you will share and discuss the reasons behind your entries. The last worksheet technique in our guide, but not the least, revolves around predicting the future of your relationship as well as letting your partner know what you want your relationship to become and how you see your relationship in the present. Divide your list into two columns, naming one of the columns Present and the other Future.

The first column should be divided into two smaller columns that should contain three wishes each.

Present		Future
Positive	Negative	
Write up all the Positive things in Your relationship you can note in the present, making a list Of three wishes About your relationship in the future	Write up all the negative things you Can note in your relationship in the present, making Three wishes on Which negative qualities you would like to see less	Make a list of three wishes regarding the Future of your relationship

CHAPTER 4 - Don't Bad-Mouth Your Spouse

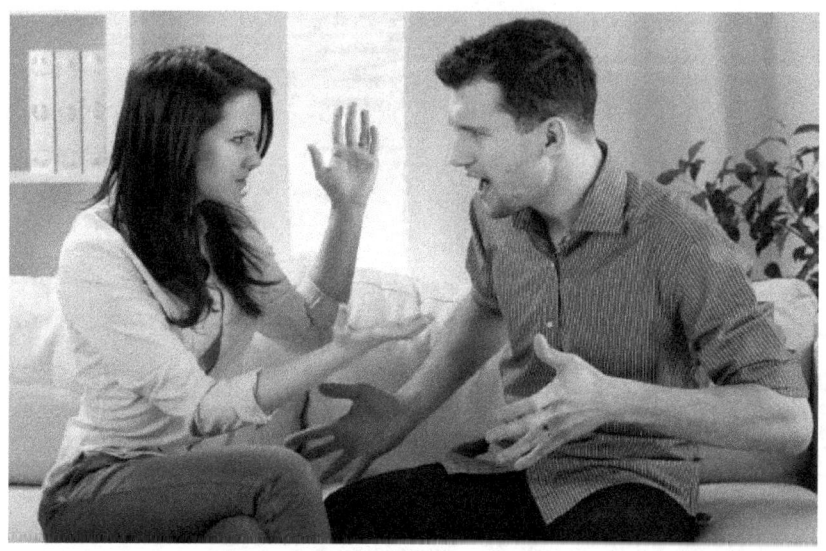

Scenario: You go out with the girls to have a few drinks, and you start talking about men. Before you know it, you're telling them about the silly things he does or that night when sex wasn't a major success (Performance issues? One of you was tired? Poor communication?). You wake up the next morning regretting the things you said, but you calm yourself down by telling yourself it was only "girl talk."

It doesn't matter whether you express a negative sentiment in front of your spouse or somebody else. Bad-mouthing your partner is never okay, and it can have long-lasting effects on the relationship.

The Dangers of Trash-Talking Your Spouse

As humans, we are all born with the tendency to gossip and complain. We make mistakes, and so do our partners. Some mistakes are easy to overlook, but others get inside the head and mess it up. They are too big to be overlooked, and thus we complain about those behaviors. To put it simply, it is impossible to live with someone and like everything about them—it just isn't going to happen.

However, how you choose to deal with this is an ever-sensitive issue we need to address. Despite knowing how effective communication between partners can resolve issues, we still avoid confiding in our spouses about the things that irk us about them. We always choose to avoid having "the talk" and instead share these complaints with others. This is very common when dealing with a spouse who repeatedly makes the same blunders over and over, and you feel like you are done with pointing it out. The frustration that builds up within you leads to dissatisfaction and unhappiness, and thus, we look to vent to someone other than them. This is where family and friends come into the picture. They become our shoulder to cry on.

Little do we know that sharing personal details about your married life with an outsider has many dangers—even when they are our parents and siblings.

If you are looking for a straightforward reason as to why you shouldn't do it, let's discuss a few.

It feels like backstabbing. If they found out that you had been bad- mouthing them behind their backs, they would feel immensely hurt, disappointed, and embarrassed. Try to imagine yourself in the same situation. How would you react if you found out that your partner had been making jokes with their friends about you and your way of doing things?

Touché, right?

Therefore, if you don't want to make them feel unvalued, unworthy, and embarrassed, you'd better focus on working out your issues together instead of complaining about them to others.

What other dangers does this bring? Let's take a look!

Secrets Get Out

Not everyone is a great secret-keeper. So, anything you say behind your partner's back may be used against you. Are you willing to take that chance and have your spouse afraid to trust you again? If they find out, they might dredge this up every time you two have a conflict. They may also hold a grudge against you, and your perfect marriage tapestry will be destroyed forever.

People Try to Fix Things

Secondly, some people, upon hearing something bad, will try to fix things for you. They may talk to your spouse to try and amend things between you two. Your spouse will be hurt that you never came to them to discuss it in the first place, and they might feel that they are not good enough. You'll need to make some hefty apologies to get things back to normal. And even if you promise your partner that you will never do it again, they won't take your word for it. They will constantly be worried about you doing it again because you did it once, and that will ruin your marriage, too. They will always feel like they are being lied to and cheated on. Trust is one of the most sacred things between couples. Are you sure you want to risk it and destroy your marriage so soon?

It Isn't Fair to Them

Third, don't forget that when you bad-mouth your spouse, you are talking about someone you live with, spend hours with, sleep with, eat with, and share a bed with. This is the person who makes your house a home. They are the ones who accompany you wherever you go and help you out with the chores. They are the ones who contribute financially and help you pay the bills on time. Instead of appreciating what they do for you, are you going to harp on the stuff they don't do with an outsider? It doesn't seem fair. Ever heard of the phrase, "don't shit where you eat?"

The Problems Become Bigger

There is also the possibility that this will lead to actual resentment between the partners. In science, there is the belief that if one keeps repeating something repeatedly, they start to believe in it. This is called visualization. It's like telling an innocent person that they murdered someone every single day, and there will come a day that they will start to believe it, too. It may take years for some, but it happens. The point is that when one of the partners chooses to talk trash about their partners with someone other than the partner themselves, they are making no effort in trying to change the situation. As they haven't communicated the issues with their partner, the spouse has no way of finding out that there is a problem, and thus keeps on doing whatever is causing the issue in the first place.

It Reinforces Negativity in A Relationship

Like visualization, it is another idea that whatever we feed our brains with, we begin to radiate and attract the same. Remember the law of attraction? Do you know how it works? When you bad-mouth your spouse over some drinks with your friends or a visit to your parent's house, you reinforce negativity. Marriage is a delicately woven thread. Negative talk is one of the many things that adds pressure and increases the chances the thread will break. The more you talk trash about your partner, the more your brain will reinforce the thoughts. Ultimately, it will become harder for you to see beyond their shortcomings, and everything about them will start to bother you.

Creates A Negative Image of Your Significant Other

Are you sure you want these people to have a negative view of your spouse in their heads? After all, they only hear one side of the story and a distorted version of it, at that. It's wrong to depict your partner negatively in the eyes of others. They will offer you terrible advice, seeing you as a victim. They will encourage you to make rash decisions that may not end well for you. What if they tell you to leave them?

Meanwhile, your spouse has no idea about what is going on and is completely unaware of the issues you hold against them. Doesn't seem too fair, does it?

It's Disrespectful

Finally, you have to admit, and it's disrespectful. Again, had you been in their position, and your spouse had done something similar, you would have felt completely unvalued and belittled. So, don't do something that will jeopardize the harmonious relationship you have. Even if you two face some minor issues, before involving a third person, try to resolve it on your own.

How to Stop Bad-Mouthing Your Spouse

This will be extremely hard, as your marriage is fairly new and everyone wants all the juicy details. They will be asking about how your sex life is, when do you plan to start a family, how is your husband/wife treating you, are they any good with the chores, etc. All these questions may not come off directly, but people will try to get some intimate details out of you no matter how much you try to remain quiet about it. And believe me, it won't be strangers or distant aunts and uncles asking for the nitty-gritty—it will be your parents, siblings, and closest friends. Saying you don't want to share or discuss the matter with them seems quite rude, doesn't it? I mean, they're your family. They worry about you. Maybe they aren't inquisitive because they need something to talk about—maybe, they're concerned about
how your partner is treating you.

So, how do you tackle such straight-forwardness and avoid bad- mouthing your spouse? Well, here are a few smart ways to go about this.

Dodge Questions About Intimacy

If you think that a relative or friend is too nosey about your sexual intimacy with your partner and you can sense what the coming questions will be like, dodge them by making up a stupid excuse like you just remembered that you had to be someplace or that you had to do something important and completely forgot. If you're at a family gathering, tell them that some aunt was calling for you and that you need to go to her. Make it believable and dodge the chance for further probing.

Talk to Your Spouse About It

If someone gives you a hard time by being rather too straightforward, let your partner know that you aren't feeling comfortable and see if they can come and rescue you from there. You can also let them know in case you did slip out some juice because they wouldn't stop investigating—that way, they won't hold it against you.

Call Them Out

In case the probing continues, and your spouse isn't around to help you out, come clean and let them know that you don't feel comfortable sharing intimate details about your relationship with anyone. It might seem rude at first, but if it is necessary, do it. This is your chance to set an unmistakable boundary and keep the follow-up questions at bay.

Use Humor to Avert the Questions

Humor is a great way to deal with difficult and nosy questions without making the asker feel bad about it. Think of it as the opposite of setting boundaries, as it keeps the situation under control and comfortable. For instance, if you're asked when you plan to start a family a hundred times by different relatives, let them know that you two are still figuring out how to do it or something equally funny as, "Well, let me check my calendar for baby-making days… Oops, it's not on the books this year."

CHAPTER 5 - Feedback: How to Give and Respond to It

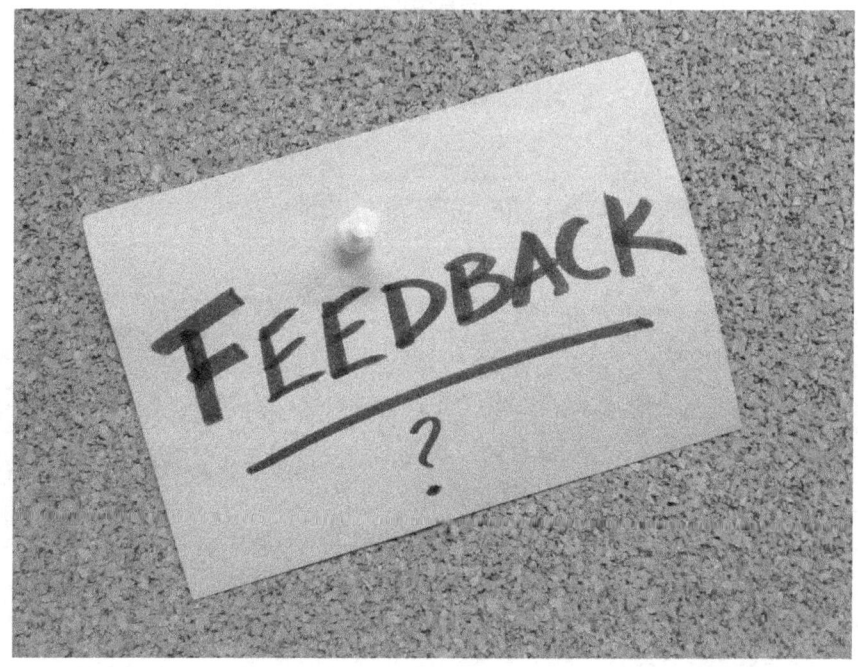

Whether we like it or not, feedback is part of our day-to-day communication. It cannot be helped that a major part of our interactions with people revolve around responding to
what they said, how they look, and what they are proposing. As such, the ability to give feedback is an essential skill to master. But an evenmore important skill is in receiving it and acting on it in the healthiestmanner possible.

Feedback and Your Brain

What exactly happens inside your head when we receive feedback? The chances are that you already feel bad for something that you did, but it is even harder to hear the same thoughts being voiced by others. And why is this so? Neuroscience tells us that the brain is designed to be a rather protective organ in the sense that it will prioritize its welfare over others, whether you are aware of it or not. In essence, it goes out of its way to protect you from negativity and make you feel that you are in the right, even if clearly, you are not.

How it works is quite simple: The brain views almost all types of feedback as criticism, and criticism, in itself, is perceived as an external threat.

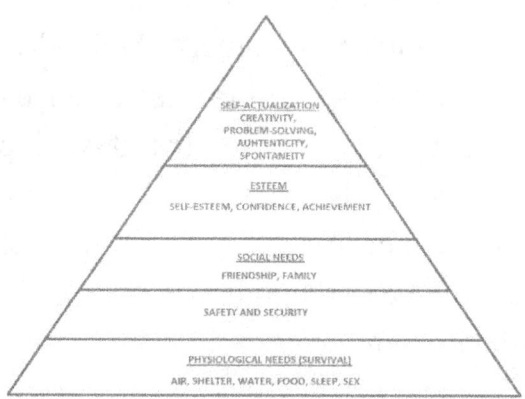

To help you understand this concept better, here's Abraham Maslow's
Hierarchy of Needs.

Generally speaking, criticism attacks the upper tiers of the hierarchy, namely self-actualization and esteem. But, for the brain, it feels like it is attacking the lower tiers (i.e., the ones primarily focused on basic survival).

Here's an example: Let us say that you had presented a report, and one of your audience members says something like, "Hey, your report had a lot of errors. I couldn't agree with what you were saying because of those."

To them, they were just saying that you need to do more research on your report before presenting it. To you, more often than not, they just attacked your very being and seemingly made your contributions to the group worthless.

One other thing about negativity is that it is retained easier on the brain but often done so inaccurately. An off-hand comment can be remembered as a serious insult or a request to do better as a personal attack depending on your mind frame in that instant.

This is what is called a negativity bias. Our brains tend to process negative feedback more than the positive but in a way that hinders proper development and communication.

Finding a workaround for this bias is important in learning how to give and receive feedback.

Offering Feedback

1. Mind Your Purpose

For what particular reason are you giving that feedback? What is your primary goal of saying something to a person who needs to hear it? Here is a list of some of the negative and positive motivations behind giving people feedback that they need to hear.

Positive	Negative
Concern for another A sense of responsibility for that person Guidance Support Encouragement Discipline	To lash out Defend or deflect your behavior To demoralize Appeasement for another party To make the person inferior

It goes without saying that the more positive motivations can result in better-worded feedback. However, just make sure that whatever feedback you give reflects that actual reason as to why you are giving it in the first place.

2. Focus on the Act, not the Actor

A crucial step to learn here is to always separate the person from hisactions. In essence, try to focus on correcting the action and not the character of the person when giving criticism. This will separate the person from the situation that they put themselves in. It's not that theyare stupid or idiotic or evil; it's just that they did something not exactly good in that instance. This way, they can focus on what you are tryingto say without being personally insulted.

3. Give a Criticism Sandwich

In essence, you give them a detailed appraisal of what just happened so that your feedback will not be seen as entirely negative.

The criticism sandwich follows this sequence:

A. Start with a positive comment

B. Focus on the strong points of the person

C. Support with complements

D. Give the criticism

E. Remind the person of their strong points

F. End on a positive note.

Let us say, for this example, that an employee of yours named Bobby went out and sealed a deal with a client without notifying you first. Perhaps you wanted to talk with that client yourself and had prepared a presentation, but one of your own just did it but without your consent.

Giving a criticism sandwich should sound like this:

"Bobby, thank you for what you did (positive comment). Had you not acted this way (strong point), we would not have sealed such a deal with that client. Thank you very much (compliment).

But next time, please notify your team or me of any interaction you will initiate with our clients. We work as a team, and we should communicate like one (criticism). But, despite that, you did good, and your initiative helped the team! (strong point)

Rest assured that our bosses and we appreciated what you did. You might even have saved your team a lot of time and money in convincing the client to close the deal. Drinks are on me tonight! (end on a positive note)."

You could even make the criticism even less stinging if you phrase it positively. Say something like "I would love if you…" or "You could do a great job if you…" or "The one thing that will make this even greater than it is if you…" If done right, you could prevent a lot of toxicity from leaking into your dialogue with that person.

Receiving Feedback

1. Build up an Immunity

What stings the most with feedback is the fact that it almost always catches us off-guard. You could prevent this by asking for feedback as often as possible, especially with the people you trust.

How you could do this is rather easy. Before you do anything, ask some open-ended questions like the following:

- If you can make two or three suggestions on how I could have done things better, what would they be?

- Is there a better way for me to handle that situation?

- Do you know of a way to make my job easier?

- If you were in my position now, would you have done things differently?

- Asking these questions frequently puts you on a direct path towards receiving feedback. As such, you tend to get less offended if people voice their concerns about you.

- On the other hand, these questions immediately put the other person in a position to add value to the conversation. They can now comment on what you did without fear of repercussions from your side.

2. Take Time to Reflect

The one thing that you shouldn't do is respond immediately to feedback. The reason for this is that humans tend to "explain away" what they did, which is seen as a rather defensive move. Let the person finish their feedback and listen intently. Once they have said their piece, reflect on what was said. You could even do multiple reflections for the same feedback before you respond to it. The goal here is to get the essence of what they are saying and what they want out of that feedback. If you understand this, your response will be more effective.

3. Embrace Your Mistakes and Grow

It is hard to admit to our mistakes, so receiving feedback is often next to impossible. More often than not, we blame our mistakes on external factors like the weather, the setup of the system, and even other people.

The idea of embracing your failures, however, has become a more prevalent concept these days. There is something so liberating and endearing with admitting that you are capable of mucking it up. And, if you do embrace your faults and mistakes, feedback that was intended to demoralize hurts less for you now.

But knowing that you make mistakes is not enough. You also have to assure you that you are working on ironing out the kinks in your personality, methodology, and any other aspect in your life that invites criticism. Once that assurance is given, all that is left to do is show that such changes are taking place.

The Bottom Line

More often than not, it is the way we provide and receive feedback that is problematic, not the content itself. Your biggest problem here will always be your perceptions. It is either you don't think too much of what the other person feels when you provide feedback or overthink the feedback you received.

This is why your barriers are the biggest hurdles you will have to clear to communicate properly. Take the time to plan what you have to say before saying them, so the person receives it in a healthy manner.

On the flip side, you also must curb your tendencies towards perceiving feedback negatively. Unless it is out in the open that that person hates the fact that you exist, do not assume negative intent for everything they throw against you. With your negativity bias dealt with, you can easily go through life without accidentally offending people by the way you interact with them or getting needlessly offended yourself

CHAPTER 6 - Kindness Is the Key to Successful Communication

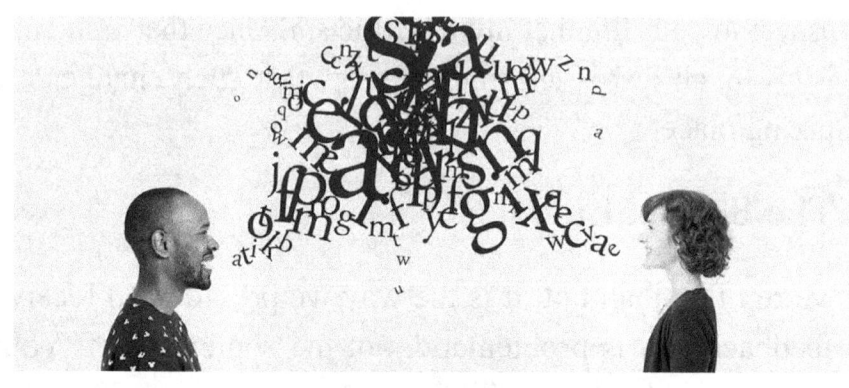

Let's distinguish between being nice and being kind. In building intimacy, being kind is essential, while being nice is often stifling.

When you are nice, you are typically (whether you are aware of it or not) thinking of the other person's feelings, adjusting what you say and how you say it to make the other person more comfortable. This means if your husband doesn't like loud noises, you don't raise your voice. If your husband might feel hurt, you don't tell him that you don't like the earrings he just gave you. It means not sharing that you didn't enjoy being touched the way he touched you last night, because it may be a blow to his ego.

I am certainly not advocating the opposite, namely focusing on yourexperience and feelings without regard to your partner's. Instead, I invite you to consider the middle ground between putting yourpartner's comfort level above all else and expressing your unfilteredinner process.

In reality, the enlightened middle ground is where real kindness resides.

When you are kind, you have your attention on your own inner experience, needs, and desires, and you also have attention on your partner's experience and how you are impacting him. When you are either being nice or being selfish, you create disconnection because you aren't honoring both of you in your communication, and being kind is fundamentally relational. Being kind also allows you to communicate with love and care. What would otherwise be hard to hear, when communicated with kindness, is much easier for whomever you are speaking to, to take in and consider.

Being kind is a concept that is fairly easy to understand but implementing it is one of the most challenging aspects of a relationship. One of the primary ways we become kind is by adjustingthe tone we use when we speak.

Very often, we are unaware of our tone and, therefore, don't realize itsimpact. If you say something to your partner and he becomes defensive, and you wonder why, evaluate your tone. The tone of voice is often how both intended and unintended feelings of criticism, dismissal, judgment, and resentment seep through. If your partner is responding as though you are unkind, it is highly likely that your tone reflects that.

When I began coaching couples, I had the privilege of experiencing them speaking with one another in ways that were not witnessed by others. Again, and again, I was somewhat shocked by how women in good, strong relationships spoke with their partners, subtly or overtly putting them down in direct communications. I also saw this in how she spoke to me about her partner, in the third person, while the three of us were in conversation in the same room together. I heard statements like:

- I'm so over how careless he is with money. It's like he's trying
to make sure our kids won't go to college.

- I'm so sick of him wearing that ugly sweatshirt. Can't you find
out how to just buy something online?

- Every day, it's the same thing with him. I'm so bored, and I practically want to fall asleep."

When I first witnessed this behavior, I was really surprised, and then I realized it was exactly how I sometimes spoke with my husband. Without observing others, I never would have recognized that my tone of voice was unkind; it seemed normal, and not the least bit noteworthy. In fact, if my husband had requested, I speak kindlier to him, I would have been certain I was already doing so.

Culturally, as empowered modern women, we are used to speaking to our male partners in ways we would never want to be spoken to ourselves. It's subtle and often easier to see our unpleasantness in hindsight rather than in the present time. Pivoting into kindness is actually quite nuanced and often more easily appreciated after the change has been made.

In practice, embracing honesty and being kind are intertwined. They are conceptually distinct, but they really need to be implemented at the same time because embracing honesty focuses on the content conveyed, and being kind focuses on the manner with which it is conveyed. Both are fundamentally necessary in order to improve communication.

Kindness is most often conveyed in our tone of voice. We can say the exact same words, but when we are unkind, we can sound derisive, judgmental, dismissive, superior, skeptical, resentful, and angry. In contrast, when we are kind, our tone can be soft, warm, humble, direct, uncomplicated, and loving. In fact, thirty percent of what we communicate is conveyed through the tone of our voices, and it's invariably the portion we are least aware of.

When a couple has a difference of opinion, it creates a recurring dynamic: Whether it is an outright disagreement or just inferred. And whether the conflict is blatant or more controlled, dramatic, or subtle, invariably, the issue is eventually put aside. You both recognize that you don't know how to move through it, and since you can't find out how to create a new resolution that works for everyone, you let it go. However, despite your best intentions to avoid the trap of an altogether familiar and painful dynamic, it eventually arises anyway. You try to avoid it, but even so, now and then, it's back, and sure enough, you both have the same emotional and intellectual positions. It feels achingly familiar and so excruciatingly mired.

Alternatively, you may be the kind of couple that processes things, talking everything through over and over. This means that once the emotional intensity of the conflict has blown over, you discuss it. You hear his side of things, and you share yours. Hours (sometimes days) later, you come to a new understanding and appreciation of one another's positions, anticipating things will feel more collaborative going forward. Then, as if you had never thoroughly worked it through, you find yourself in an almost identical dynamic the next time the issue arises. Maybe it's a little simpler the next time because you know where your partner is coming from, and maybe it's a little worse because you both know where the other is coming from and can use that against each other. Either way, processing helps mitigate things after the fact and get to know one another better, but it doesn't actually prevent the conflict from recurring.

The problem with processing is that understanding is rarely enough to create new behavior. This is why you have probably experienced having a conflict, processing it, only to find yourself in the same conflict again, feeling as though you never worked it through. This cycle is frustrating and sometimes paves the way back to the first scenario, where you just let the issue go because talking about it ultimately feels futile, and it's too frustrating to feel that way.

Happily, there is an excellent way to break this cycle; there is another alternative besides avoidance and analysis. Instead, you can create new experiences that are wholesome and harmonious, innovative and honest, by doing what I describe as a conscious redo. The conscious redo is designed to form new ways of feeling, communicating, and acting mid-conflict; you can access new experiences and never have to go back and relive the same frustrations again. The dictionary definition of redo is "to do something again, especially to do it better." The potency of this tool comes from using it repeatedly. Each time you use it, you will become more skillful with it, eventually learning to employ it right in the middle of the conflict, while you are literally in the heat of the moment.

Instead of processing and understanding, and having a Deja vu experience as you start the conflict all over again, you stop and redo your communications at the moment. You make a conscious choice to create a new experience that is more satisfying for both of you. From a neurological perspective, it means that you create new neural pathways in response to the same trigger, instead of firing the same pathways again and again. This results in the formation of new habits while amid intense emotions. The result is freedom from the compulsion of the familiar dynamic, and the creativity to interact more productively.

A successful conscious redo requires a lot of awareness in both of you and courage and the willingness to be vulnerable. It takes practice to become aware while feeling activated, internally create enough space to take a short time out, regroup, and then proceed in a new and improved, much kinder way. This is a learnable skill, and with practice comes the ability to participate in successful conscious redos.

When you have the desire to apologize for what you said or how you said it, when you find yourself in a familiar dynamic that you don't enjoy, when you feel insulted, attacked, or otherwise disrespected by your partner, these are all moments to disrupt the dynamic. Pause for a moment and request a conscious redo.

Either one of you can request the conscious redo, whether you want to redo how you have spoken, or you want to redo how you were spoken to. Initially, it is common for the person who is spoken to in an unkind way to recognize that redo is necessary. With practice, you may find yourself becoming much more conscious of both how you feel and how you speak. When you don't like how you feel or sound, you can request a conscious redo because you want to practice showing up more lovingly in your relationship, and you want both you and your partner to feel that painful interactions can be alchemized.

It doesn't matter who makes the request. Either way, the one who didn't make the request always has full permission to say yes, no, or not yet. If the requested partner isn't ready, wait until a better time and then proceed with the conscious redo, starting from just before the communications became problematic. If a person doesn't want to do a conscious redo, it is often because the person is so angry or otherwise distraught that they can't access another way of communicating at that moment. In this case, it is best to take a true intermission in the conversation and wait to return to it once both people can be present, non-reactive, and can choose how they behave.

Sometimes one partner requests a conscious redo, and the other partner doesn't know what to adjust because it felt fine the first time. In that scenario, the partner who requested the conscious redo should state as simply as possible what was unpleasant for them. It is important to describe your own experience rather than blaming your partner for doing something wrong.

CHAPTER 7 - Grow Together

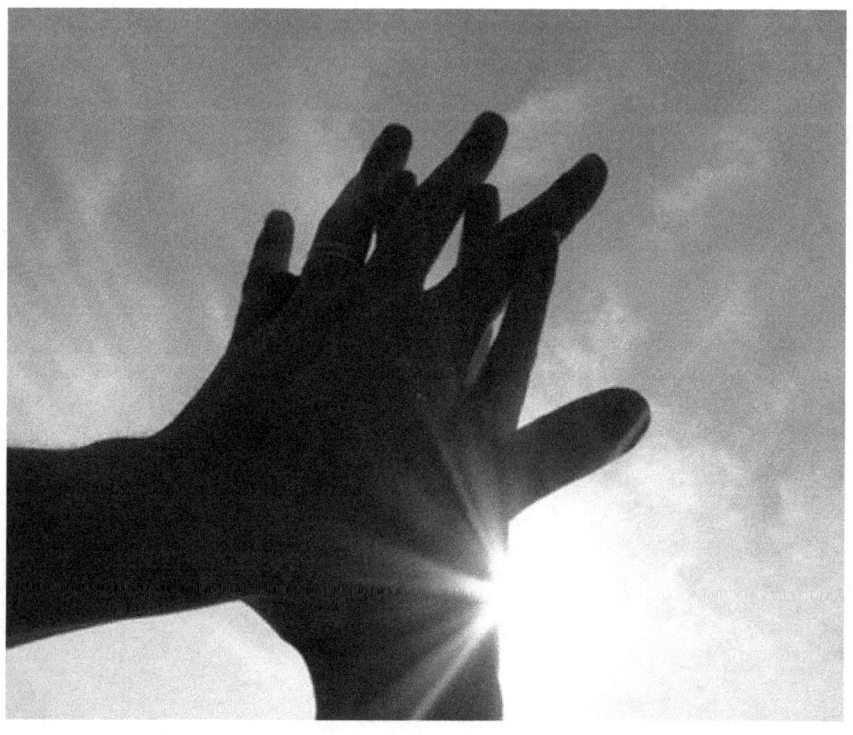

You should make it your priority to evolve together, expecting each other in difficult times continually. Good communication is the key when it comes to growing together. Good
communication involves spouses showing each other that they are listening. Having a conversation with someone who is utterly quiet can make one feel conversing with themselves.

It is, therefore, important that every spouse contributes to show they are listening. For example, a spouse may add on to what the other person has said. This shows that everyone is listening attentively and processing the issues. If, for example, one person is talking about their day at work, the partner may say, "It sounds as if that office has some people with personal issuers rubbing off on everybody. The things that the secretary said would tick me off too." The person may also add, "What can I do to make your day better." Language like this shows a partner that they have been understood and that they can get help if they need it.

Good communication is not all about talking and talking. Sometimes, the best medicine involves a good level of silence. For instance, when two people have a conversation, they can take a break to digest what they have said to each other. The silence will help the two people put their thoughts in order and avoid blurting out things unintentionally. Open communication and conversation do not mean going on and on in an endless conversation. Take a break and a breath. Good silence also indicates to the partners that they are reflecting on all that has been said.

Good and open communication requires one to be sensitive to the moods, schedules, and other factors of their partner. Select a good time to have an effective back and forth based on the conversation you want to have. However, things that need to be addressed should not be ousted too far off. Address matters openly as soon as possible because dwelling on them in silence will bring problems. One should pick a suitable moment as soon as possible and open up.

Another important factor that can help couples grow together is honoring the opinions of a partner even if they differ. Honoring different views is one of the main keys to good communication. To show honor of different opinions, one may say, "I understand what you are saying, but I think... Can we agree to disagree?" Such statements will not only acknowledge that one person has understood the other but also that they respect a different opinion. They also help one state their different opinion without overstepping their boundaries. Honoring the views of each other de-escalates what could have become a conflict.

Couples need to identify ways of having the most productive conversations, which will add value to their marriage. One of the best ways of maintaining an emotional connection is through holding good open conversations. Couples should segregate time to hold conversations and put some of the tips named above into practice.

The Importance of Practicing Day After Day to Achievea Mindful Relationship

Communication in marriage and connection are directly related. Without one, the other is likely to fail. When people express themselves adequately, things tend to be better even when they cannotagree on a particular subject. For instance, if a couple is talking abouthow much money they should spend on entertainment per month, they may want more to go to movies and games while the wife wants more to go with her girlfriends for shopping sprees. The couple maynot initially agree on the amount they should spend, but so long as they communicate about it, they both understand what the other wants. When communication is a challenge, one may feel that the other is being wasteful and still not express it in the right way. Bad communication leads to feelings of isolation, sadness, loneliness, heartbroken, and disheartened. Communication is important for both simple and tough reasons. In the movies, couples seem to have some almost perfect lives, but in thereal world, it is more complicated than that. People have to decide about children, money, work-life, obligations, and other action itemswithout a screen script to follow. Such matters call on the couples tohave deep conversations. Even the little things that could be ignored before the couple lives together have to be taken into consideration; otherwise, the marriage might fail. Without the right communication in marriage, drifts happen, and the couple that was ones so in love becomes strangers sharing a table. Again, communication in marriage differs from communication in a relationship because couples tend to get tired of the masks want to deal with real feelings. The spouses want to be heard; their deep needs start to surface; they want to be validated. If one person keeps dismissing, interrupting, or shutting down their partner, there will be a rift between them.

Good communication leads to a great marriage and more. As seen earlier, communication and connection go together, and consequently, if one goes down, the other fails. Every couple should strive to revive the communication whenever there are hiccups because it will lead to stronger intimacy both physically and emotionally. Communication is not required in marriage just for emotional and physical connection. The couples also need to make decisions about development and growth.

In many cases, development and growth involve making decisions about the money. When two people come together in marriage, there are many emotions that get tied up in how they spend money. If the couple keeps pushing aside conversations about money decisions, a lot of problems will arise soon in the family. Communication is also important because people only have a finite amount of time on earth-no one wants to be in a relationship where there is no connection. That is why many people opt for divorces when the spouses are no longer connected. One way to avoid separations and stay connected for a long time is to keep rediscovering things about one another more so through communication. Change for the better and show it to one another that you are putting effort into working. Share experiences, create new memories that you can discuss later, and laugh. Good communication ensures that the couple knows which statements would make the other person shut down or build a wall; therefore, they avoid offending one another. Good communication is proactive such that, instead of waiting for things to go wrong to start a conversation, the couple sorts things out in time. The results of goodcommunication are a solid foundation in the marriage where the couple can talk about anything without fear.

Many couples who have communication difficulties think that it will take an arm and a leg to get back on track. Although this might be true for some broken communications, most couples need to make small steps towards better communication, and they will achieve a considerable difference. A few adjustments to the channels of communication, and the spouses will achieve a tremendous compounding effect on their relationship and marriage. While facing communication challenges, many couples also tend to feel like they are the only ones undergoing this. They need to remember that they are not the only ones facing challenges. Challenges are normal in every relationship. The key to solving the problems is consistency.

Remember, a distance between couples or any two people does not happen overnight. There is not just one reason which leads to a total drift in a couple that was once madly in love. It results from small omissions and commissions that offend the other person, therefore, creating mountains of differences and gaps between the two people. In the initial stages of a relationship and marriage, a couple can easily thrive on excitement and physical attraction, therefore, communication plays a small role, and many of its aspects will be ignored.

As the bond between the two individuals deepens, the attraction changes very fast into the first stages of love, where every person is making a foundation of trust. This is because they want to have a stronger and happier future. When in marriage, the love that once thrived on attraction and excitement changes to one that is sustained by trust, commitment, and honesty. Over the years, the responsibilities change, and the amount of stress increases with an increase in challenges. Somehow, the time to be there for one another and to share seems to diminish.

Communication becomes a chore that couples would rather skip even if it is talking about a joyous moment. Things seem to change, and the couples that thought marriage is a completely smooth ride usually feel cheated or lost. The suppressed negative feelings that arise from this situation make a couple preys to miscommunication or total lack of it. Then the drift occurs, followed by assumption and mistrusts, in worse cases, infidelity, lack of respect, dishonesty, etc. Good communication means that a couple respects one another enough to stay honest.

Demystifying the Fairytales

In all healthy relationships, communication must act as the centerpiece. All individuals in all relationships, whether in marriage or workplace, must maintain good communication and check in regularly. Marriages consist of more than just keeping a household, parenting, and taking care of bills. With time, the couple begins to understand that the fairy tale- happily ever after has many holes, and it takes a lot of effort from both sides to make it work.

In real life, knights on horses rarely ride in and rescue damsels in distress to a happily ever after situation. Consequently, spouses need to remember to talk to one another rather than at each other. Married Couples are in a full-time job called marriage, where they should always love and appreciate each other to achieve their marriage goals. The difficult part is that most spouses in marriages do not know how to alter their mentality to accommodate real-life things that make marriages work. That is why when many couples have difficulties communicating; they focus on the divorce statistics and the number of maintenance cases in the courts. When the spouses realize that the number of cases is too high, they get into panic mode and set the same expectations for their own homes. These expectations and standards tend to kill the marriages that would otherwise thrive. It is wrong for people to use what is happening around them to gauge their marriages. Most of the statists given to the public only involve detrimental unions. They hardly tell people of the winning marriages and how they got there. In other words, those offering statistics to the public do not tell them what it takes for the marriages to fail or succeed. They fail to discuss the satisfaction levels and communication in marriages, and therefore people do not realize that most marriages fail because of things that would be solved through communication.

CHAPTER 8 - Understanding the Impact of Trauma

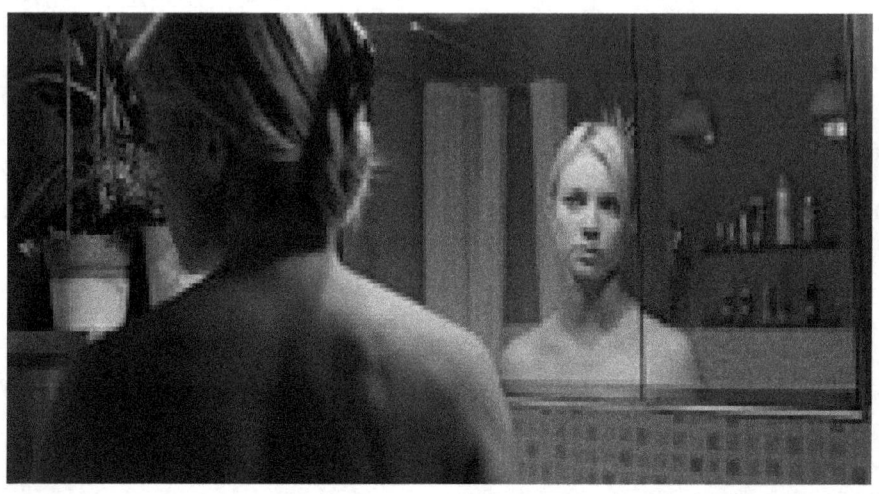

Trauma is defined as a deeply distressing or disturbing experience. Experienced trauma can have you reliving or rethinking the event over and over again in your mind due to
the damage that took hold in your soul. So, for your soul to go through this type of pain, you may have had to deal with some events, such as rape, abandonment, loss of a loved one, and molestation, which leads to identity issues and to hurt felt images in mind.

Some type of trauma could have your soul deeply wounded, like a broken cistern of living water, flowing right out of you. Have you ever noticed times when you are reading the word, but nothing is sticking? This is because your soul has open holes of damage, and the living water is flowing out instead of rushing through you. For the Word of God to flow, the soul has to be sealed with the Word of God, allowing Him to feel those cracks of the broken soul.

When we look at the soul, we look at it as part of the science that makes up the body. You are made up of 3 beings, which are the soul, mind, and Spirit. The Spirit is the direct communication to God; the soul is what goes to heaven or hell, and the mind is the connection between the Spirit and the soul. From the flow of the thoughts, you can tell where the damage state of the soul is located. When your soul is damaged, the Spirit and mind cannot flow how God wants it to flow. Let us say God wants to use you prophetically by the power of the Holy Ghost, but your soul is damaged. All you can receive is a bad transmitter, and you cannot flow thoroughly in the gift of that Spirit.

Different types of trauma can cause the soul to become damaged, depending on the event that happened. When a person is molested or raped, the event can cause a lot of trauma to the soul because the soul becomes sick, and the person replays the event repeatedly in their mind.

Tamar was David's daughter by Maacah. It is important to know the back story of how David received his wife, Maacah. He got with her out of spite with King Saul. King Saul was very jealous of King David, due to the victories that David received. They had a song about them, "King Saul slays thousands, but King David 10 thousand." When King Saul heard this, he became afraid of King David. Since King

Saul wasagainst King David, David married his wife.

Now look closely at this dysfunction. Tamar was conceived out of envy and rage. When your soul is not healed, you end up passing down an unhealed soul, instead of a healed and whole, healthy soul. There was no connection with King David and Maacah, other than they were together out of anger. These emotions were passed through the bloodline of trauma.

Later, Tamar was raped by her brother, Amon, who was her half- brother. They had different mothers, but King David was their father. The bible states Amon became sick over his sister. His soul was in turmoil over having his sister in the bed. Once his soul became sick, he thought about her day and night, lusting over his sister. As he becamesick in the soul and mind, his body starting craving Tamar.

One day, while he was becoming ill over Tamar, his cousin came up to him and asked why a King was looking so sick? He went on to tell him the desire he had over his sister. What is so powerful about this is theSpirit on Amon knew who to come to for the plan to be carried out.

See, we attach to whom we are in the Spirit within us. We stick to spirits of our brokenness or our healing. So, this Spirit came to Amonto carry out this act. The cousin told Amon to pretend as if he was sick, physically. So, Amon went to tell his dad to send for his sister, Tamar, to cook for him. King David sent Tamar up to the room. When she came into the room, Amon tricked her and told her to come near and feed him. Once Tamar got close to him, he attacked her viciously. She said to him, let us get married. She was attempting to prevent the trauma of the soul; however, he attacked her anyway. Once he was done attacking her, he threw her out of the room.

After Tamar was raped, she left the room with deep sorrow. In those days, a sign of being in deep mourning was to put ashes on your face and rip your clothing. Tamar was deeply distressed, so she ripped her clothes off, due to the deep feeling of unworthiness. She was a virgin waiting for her husband, but instead, her innocence was taken. She did not feel that she was worthy to ever be used. We never heard anything about Tamar again.

Let us break down this trauma of the soul: Rejection & Abandonment

King David never came and helped his daughter from her pain. King David was too hurt and caught up in the pain of losing a child, and now his daughter was raped. Tamar felt rejected and abandoned. She feels unworthy because Amon did not want to marry her, but he wanted her purified body. Once the soul has endured this type of pain, the mind begins to develop thoughts of defeat and discouragement, which cause us to act out on rejection and unworthiness, making us walk in pity and not power and causes us to walk in a false identity, the identity God did not give you.

God did not give us the Spirit of fear; abuse makes you walk in fear, which is a false part of your identity in God. Fear is a pity and makes you a person full of shame and condemnation, fearing that people will find out what you are going through.

Most people who have experienced molestation try their hardest to keep it as a secret. This is not the person, but the Spirit in operation, trying to keep them from exposing the secret. Once the secret is released, there is no longer any power over you. By keeping the experience as a secret, the enemy has the full power of their family. But when you stand up and tell the secret, restoration and healing take place for their family. If you can control the abuse in your life, then walk away with the power of knowing God has you. If fear arises, then walk out anyway. The enemy will come with fear to make you forfeit what God is truly saying to keep you in cycles.

The Trauma of the Abuse

Abuse is defined as a bad effect or for an evil purpose—misuse. For years, I allowed my life to be in the hands of a man who misused my body; the purpose of our relationship was misuse. We misuse each other's body, our minds, and traumatized our souls. Everyone has a purpose, but sometimes we misuse the body for a purpose God did not design for us.

God designed our bodies to be His temple to dwell in us, but unfortunately, we crave the things of this world and end up misusing the purpose of our bodies. We use our bodies for our selfish desires, sex, drugs, and the use of the world. God designed sex for marriage as a reward for being in covenant. Like a weapon towards the enemy, God uses it as a war tactic against the enemy. However, when our little minds get exposed to something of this world, we do not know the value or purpose for our bodies, and we end up feeding our bodies what it was not made to have. We were called to live a holy and blameless life before God, but instead, we use our life for our purpose.

When we end up using our bodies for our gratifications of the world, we cause mistreat to settle in. When we drive our bodies to go through trauma, we are pushing our souls and minds to go through abuse. We become too damaged to love again and allow the damage to keep us from trusting again. We allow our bodies to be used, and when our bodies are misused, we cause damage to our soul, which prevents us from walking into our full power. Instead, we assume a false power, which is not much when your damaged goods, and you feel as damaged goods, lead you into thinking you do not have the ability to walk it out.

We become too damaged to walk in power because when we misuse our bodies, we incorrectly program ourselves and end up craving the opposite of what the Spirit wants. We cause identity issues by allowing the blow of words, or the blow of hands, to mistreat our bodies and minds. We put our souls in danger of not understanding the agape love God has for us. Agape love is the highest a person can offer. This love is understanding, compassionate, slow to anger; this love is not tangible; it is a love that only God can give; however, when your love has been mistreated due to mind and body misuse, the dangers leave holes in your soul that can't process this type of love. Rather than recognizing love, a damaged soul only understands hate, and it has a lack of understanding, it is fault-finding, has a sense of unworthiness, and lacks confidence; which in all, puts us in danger to crave these things and attracts the same types of people.

A damaged soul puts you in danger of having these types of people coming into your life, time after time, and you won't understand why you keep attracting the same kind of people. You will keep attracting toxic people, abusive men, men who only want to use you, who have no self-esteem, can't keep a job, have any stability, and no potential to ever marry you. You keep attracting them because of the mistreatment and trauma of your body and soul. You are attracting them because this is what you think you deserve, and you have programmed your mind to believe this is all you can earn and all you would get.

CONCLUSION

When a mother gives birth, when the baby cries, it is a normal situation that reflects a new life. This cry reflects the cycle of life, representing the greatest amount of a person's emotions regarding joy, pain, grief and pain. As part of life, we usually love someone who we think is the right one for us. Falling in love is the greatest emotion that words cannot understand. It's a wonderful feeling, a genuine joy that stimulates our senses to think and do things for ourselves for someone we love. If we fall in love, we feel something weird, and it's a great feeling, it's a complete joy in life to be with someone we love. If someone you love isn't your true partner in life, things will happen so fast that your hopes will be broken, your feelings will be cut off, and your heart will break. It is then that moment when you experience the pain of a broken heart and change your thoughts and feelings. With this book I wanted to help you make your relationship a safe place without anxiety and without the risk of attacks from your partner, to live your relationship in peace.
Good luck.

CPSIA information can be obtained
at www.ICGtesting.com
Printed in the USA
LVHW080144230521
688251LV00002B/126